YOUR KNOWLEDGE HAS VALUE

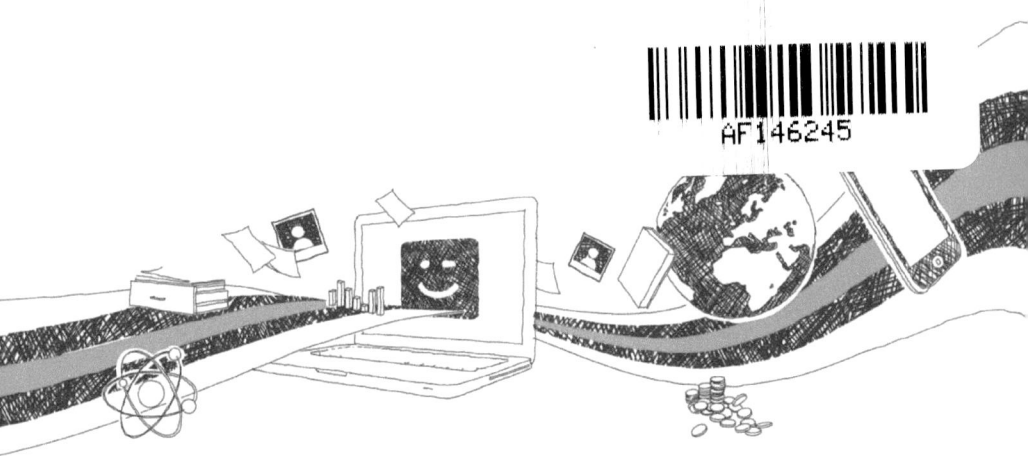

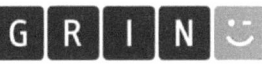

Bibliographic information published by the German National Library:

The German National Library lists this publication in the National Bibliography; detailed bibliographic data are available on the Internet at http://dnb.dnb.de .

Imprint:

Copyright © 2017 GRIN Verlag, Open Publishing GmbH
Print and binding: Books on Demand GmbH, Norderstedt Germany
ISBN: 9783668419049

This book at GRIN:

http://www.grin.com/en/e-book/355067/the-weight-loss-effects-of-an-lchf-diet-a-statistical-meta-analysis-of

Robert Stewart

The Weight Loss Effects of an LCHF Diet. A Statistical Meta-Analysis of Meta-Analyses

GRIN Publishing

GRIN - Your knowledge has value

Since its foundation in 1998, GRIN has specialized in publishing academic texts by students, college teachers and other academics as e-book and printed book. The website www.grin.com is an ideal platform for presenting term papers, final papers, scientific essays, dissertations and specialist books.

Visit us on the internet:

http://www.grin.com/

http://www.facebook.com/grincom

http://www.twitter.com/grin_com

The Weight Loss Effects of an LCHF Diet:

A Statistical Meta-Analysis of Meta-Analyses

DHSC 9055 Applied Research Project

Robert W. Stewart

A.T. Still University

A course assignment presented to the College of Graduate Health Studies in partial fulfillment of the requirements for the Doctor of Health Science Degree A.T. Still University

February 15th, 2017

Abstract

Given the existing problem of obesity, the purpose of this statistical meta-analysis was to measure the weight-loss effectiveness of LCHF diets. Using Cohen's d as the measure, it was found that the mean effect size for LCHF diets was higher ($M = 0.5333$, $SD = 0.29209$) than the mean effect size for non-LCHF diets at an Alpha of 0.10, $p = 0.058$. Additionally, it was found that the mean effect size for LCHF diets ($M = 0.5333$, $SD = 0.29209$) in comparison to control (non-diet) groups ($M = 0.0358$, $SD = 0.03470$), $p < 0.001$ was also higher. These findings provide empirical support for the claim that LCHF diets are effective, both in isolation and in comparison to other dietary interventions.

Keywords: LCHF, low carbohydrate high fat, obesity, weight loss.

Content

The Weight Loss Effects of an LCHF Diet: A Statistical Meta-Analysis of Meta-Analyses

Obesity has been described as a premier public health problem in developed countries, America in particular (Frederick, Snellman, & Putnam, 2014; Karp et al., 2014; Kay & McLaughlin, 2014; Zilanawala et al., 2015; Zukiewicz-Sobczak et al., 2014). Obesity has been demonstrated to play a causal role in the development of many ailments, including cardiovascular disease and diabetes. Public health authorities, policy-makers, scientists, non-profit and for-profit businesses around the world have made attempts to reduce the obesity problem by recommending modifications of diet to the members of their communities'. In the United States, awareness of the need to consciously manipulate diet to protect against obesity dates from the 19th century, when the increasing availability of calories and the decreasing need for physical labor indicated the beginning of a major shift in the body mass index (BMI) of Americans (Kaplan, Hill, Lancaster, & Hurtado, 2000). However, for well over a century, there has been continuous and contentious scholarly dispute over the effectiveness of specific diets (Zuk, 2013).

A low-carbohydrate, high-fat (LCHF) diet has been practiced in many settings. There is some evidence that an LCHF diet was the cornerstone of aboriginal diets in many regions (including Canada, Alaska, and Scandinavia) in which fat from animals was a more readily available source of calories (Fumagalli et al., 2015; Thorburn, Macia, & Mackay, 2014). In contemporary settings different iterations of the LCHF diet have been adopted by individuals, either on the basis of scientific recommendations or as a selective return to alleged ancestral eating patterns (Zuk, 2013).

Background

Despite the existence of empirical studies on the effectiveness of an LCHF diet, specifically the effectiveness of LCHF diets (in terms of weight loss) this is limited in regards to retrospective analyses. The absence of retrospective reviews of the effectiveness of LCHF diets could mean that additional evidence could be realized about the effectiveness of such diets, especially in comparison to other diets. The opportunity for performing this meta-analysis is to gain a better understanding of the effects of an LCHF diet on weight loss through the synthetization of prior LCHF research data.

Purpose of the Study

The purpose of this study is to measure the weight-loss effectiveness of LCHF diets by conducting a meta-analysis of meta-analyses, to test the strength of prior evidence gathered.

3

This purpose will be achieved in two ways. First, the effect size of LCHF diets on weight loss will be calculated in isolation. Second, the effect size of LCHF diets on weight loss will be compared to the effect sizes of other kinds of diets on weight loss. The findings will thus offer two complementary measures, relative and absolute, of the weight-loss effectiveness of LCHF diets.

Study Design and Methods

Scholars have long called attention to the superior reliability of meta-analyses. The theory of statistical meta-analysis is based on the central claim that the pooled average of multiple effect sizes is superior to a single study's reported effect size (Cochrane, 1972). One specific advantage of meta-analytical pooling is that effect sizes can be given different weights based on the quality of the studies from which they are derived; thus, for example, more weight can be ascribed to results based on the level of evidence they display (Campbell, 1988; Cochrane, 1972). LCHF diets and weight loss are particularly appropriate for statistical meta-analysis because of the existence of a large number of existing studies on this topic. Therefore, instead of attempting to generate new primary research on the relationship between LCHF diets and weight loss, it is more expedient to pool existing research to derive a measure of effect size. Thus a retrospective review and analysis of meta-analyses to identify effectiveness of LCHF diets was performed.

To proceed from information to knowledge, it is necessary, first of all, to define what the information is. In terms of the effects of LCHF on weight loss, there are many different results in the empirical literature and therefore a necessity for scholars to make sense of these results in a manner that can inform practice and scholarship. By sorting through existing information to reach a single, more reliable conclusion, statistical meta-analysis plays an important role in providing a transition from information to knowledge.

Research Question

A research question for a statistical meta-analysis ought to be based on a population, intervention, comparator, and outcomes (PICO) approach (Dickson & Cherry, 2014). In existing studies of diets and weight loss, there is substantial variation in PICO components. In terms of population, some studies sample children or adolescents (Pulgaron, E. R., & Delamater, A. M. (2014); whereas, others sample adults (Soltani, S., Shirani, F., Chitsazi, M. J., & Salehi-Abargouei, A. (2016). In terms of the intervention, there is variability in terms of (a) how the diets effects are measured and (b) how the diets are defined. In some studies (Peters, H. P., Bouwens, E. C., Schuring, E. A., Haddeman, E., Velikov, K. P., & Melnikov, S. M. (2014), only the effect of one kind of diet is measured; in other studies (Tonstad, S.,

Malik, N., & Haddad, E. (2014), the effects of several different kinds of diets are compared. In addition, researchers have defined diets in different ways, for example, in terms of calories below maintenance or the macronutrient composition percentages of LCHF diets. Weight loss is a common outcome measurement, but so is change in body fat percentage and change in body mass index (BMI).

The research question for this study is a synthesis of questions asked by previous studies. Specifically, this study asks: "what is the effect of an LCHF diet on weight loss among non-hospitalized American adults as measured after a minimum of 6 months?"

Literature Review

Physiology does not provide a complete theoretical account of the relationship between diets and weight loss, for the reason that different dietary approaches affect calorie consumption in other ways. While physiology provides the underlying theoretical foundation—often abbreviated CICO, or Calories In, Calories Out—quantifying the relationship between calorie consumption and weight loss, physiology alone does not explain why, for instance, some diets have a higher rate of compliance than that of others (Chambers, McCrickerd, & Yeomans, 2015; Faith, Heo, Kral, & Sherry, 2013; Halford & Harrold, 2012; Poulsen et al., 2014; Westerterp-Plantenga, Lemmens, & Westerterp, 2012). More specific biological theories must therefore be brought forward to investigate LCHF diets, or, indeed, any diet (Cooper, Stevenson, & Paton, 2016; Gibbons et al., 2013; Gluck, Yahav, Hashim, & Geliebter, 2014; Hill, Rolls, Roe, De Souza, & Williams, 2013; Jaremka et al., 2015; Sarker, Franks, & Caffrey, 2013).

Macronutrient- and Micronutrient-Related Effects

Switching to an LCHF diet has other effects that can also have an influence on the trajectory of weight loss. One possible influence involves the role of the macronutrient of protein. If an LCHF diet is adopted as part of a purposive weight loss plan, then it is highly likely that some of the missing carbohydrate calories will be replaced by protein (Westerterp-Plantenga et al., 2012). As a macronutrient, protein has a more satiating effect than either carbohydrates or fat. In addition, protein has a higher metabolic cost, that is, a higher percentage of calories expended in the attempt to digest and process protein. Some estimates suggest that only 80-85% of protein calories are stored, with the remaining 10-15% of protein calories expended in processing (Mitchell et al., 2015; Schneider, 2013). By contrast, sugar and simple carbohydrates are processed remarkably efficiently and quickly. Thus, isocaloric protein-only and carbohydrate-only meals would have different impacts on body composition, as perhaps 80-85 calories of the protein meal, but 95%-97% calories of the carbohydrate meal, would be absorbed by the body.

Thus, one of the benefits of an LCHF diet is the transference of formerly carbohydrate calories into protein calories. Assuming that an LCHF diet is also a higher-protein diet, each gram of protein that replaces each gram of carbohydrate would result in roughly 0.5 fewer net calories absorbed by the body (Mitchell et al., 2015; Schneider, 2013). If a dieter on an LCHF template were to replace 100 grams of carbohydrate with 100 grams of protein, but keep his or her diet isocaloric, he or she would thereby store 50 fewer calories a day—a trivial amount, but one that, over a year, represents 5.2 pounds of bodyweight.

The inefficient nature of protein digestion is a boon to the LCHF dieter who replaces carbohydrates with protein. However, given protein's satiety effects (Westerterp-Plantenga et al., 2012), the inevitable increase of protein following a reduction in carbohydrate is likely to reduce calorie consumption even further. Thus, one intriguing mechanism for the weight loss effectiveness of an LCHF could be such a diet's subsequent association with increased protein consumption.

Reducing carbohydrates could also benefit weight loss through the mechanism of nutritional sufficiency. People with high-carbohydrate diets, particularly as consumed in the United States, include substantial amount of simple carbohydrates in their diets. These simple carbohydrates are nutritionally empty. Therefore, no matter how many such grams of carbohydrate are consumed, the body continues to experience a depletion of certain micronutrients and vitamins, which in turn triggers hunger signals. This phenomenon has been described as the intersection of obesity and malnutrition (Horvath, de Castro, Kops, Malinoski, & Friedman, 2014; Panagopoulou, Fotoulaki, Nikolaou, & Nousia-Arvanitakis, 2014; Prentice, 2006; Tanumihardjo et al., 2007; Wells, 2012, 2013; Zapatero et al., 2013). As obese individuals might have low quantities of certain micronutrients and vitamins, their brains might continue to send out hunger signals in the hope a body will consume these micronutrients and vitamins (Horvath et al., 2014; Panagopoulou et al., 2014; Prentice, 2006; Tanumihardjo et al., 2007; Wells, 2012, 2013; Zapatero et al., 2013).

Among people who adopt an LCHF diet, one natural outcome is the reduction of calories from simple carbohydrates, which, in theory, would prime the body to seek out and consume micronutrients and vitamins from other sources, such as complex carbohydrates. Because complex carbohydrates are lower in calories than isovoluminous amounts of simple carbohydrates, it is likely that they will be featured more prominently in LCHF diets. Once individuals who substitute complex carbohydrates for simple carbohydrates, they are likely to consume more necessary micronutrients and vitamins, which, in turn, will improve satiety. Moreover, the satiety effect of the switch to a greater volume of complex carbohydrates is complemented by the satiety of a higher-protein diet. Thus, there are likely to be positive and complementary effects of micronutrient and macronutrient profile changes brought on by an LCHF diet.

One fascinating aspect of nutritional science is the stark divergence between the laws of physiology that underlie CICO and the immense variability in how humans respond to diets. While all diets will yield weight loss if they follow the CICO principle (Crino et al., 2015; Hopkins et al., 2016; Phillips, 2014; Thomas et al., 2014; Thomas et al., 2013; Weijenberg et al., 2013; Wells, 2013), not all diets are as easy to maintain. The review of findings from the literature indicated that there are three main mechanisms by which LCHF diets might be more readily associated with fat loss. First, LCHF diets might promote satiety through the added consumption of animal fats and fiber from complex carbohydrates (Berti et al., 2015; Fallaize et al., 2013; Gibbons et al., 2016). Second, LCHF diets might promote a switch to a fat-burning metabolism associated with reduced water and glycogen weight as well as with the depletion of stored body fat (Berti et al., 2015; Fallaize et al., 2013; Gibbons et al., 2016). Third, LCHF diets might result in an increased consumption of protein and also micronutrients from complex carbohydrates, both of which could help to decrease hunger signals and thereby promote weight loss or weight management (Horvath et al., 2014; Panagopoulou et al., 2014; Prentice, 2006; Tanumihardjo et al., 2007; Wells, 2012, 2013; Zapatero et al., 2013). Cumulatively, these reasons suggest that LCHF diets have multiple, complementary ways to promote a long-term energy imbalance as a result of which stored body fat can be metabolized.

Method Search

A search is a preliminary search of the literature on a meta-analytical topic (Dickson & Cherry, 2014; Dundar & Fleeman, 2014; Torgerson, 2004). Scoping searches are followed by a more detailed description of how identified studies were culled for purposes of meta-analysis (Dickson & Cherry, 2014; Dundar & Fleeman, 2014; Torgerson, 2004). In this section, both the search and the more detailed study selection processes have been discussed. The search was conducted on MEDLINEEMBASE, and the Cochrane Library Database of Clinical Trials. The following provides a couple examples of the search strings used: "weight loss" AND "low-carbohydrate, high fat" and "fat loss" AND "low-carbohydrate, high fat". The complete list of search strings that were used can be found in Appendix A.

These results were used to identify the initial studies loaded into the PRISMA flow Diagram. The PRISMA flow diagram presented in Figure 1 outlines the entire process of study selection for the statistical meta-analysis, beginning from the records identified through the scoping search and continuing through to the selection of the 12 studies included in the meta-analysis. It should be noted that the inclusion of 10-15 high-quality and relevant sources is considered acceptable in statistical meta-analysis (Dickson & Cherry, 2014; Dundar & Fleeman, 2014; Torgerson, 2004).

In the PRISMA diagram located in Appendix B, it should be noted that an effort was made to identify relevant studies that were not meta-analyses. This effort was undertaken because the number of recent meta-analyses of LCHF effects on weight loss appeared to be somewhat low. Ultimately, only three non-meta-analyses were included in the meta-analysis. The inclusion of these non-meta-analytical studies raised the quality of the meta-analysis, as, without them, there would have been only nine studies included.

Data Analysis

Perhaps the common element of statistical meta-analyses is the testing of effect size (McGraw & Wong, 1992; Rosenthal, 1994; Thalheimer & Cook, 2002). However, there are many ways to calculate effect size. Even the effect sizes reported in a study are likely to represent one of several alternate ways in which effect sizes can be calculated (Thalheimer & Cook, 2002). One common measure of effect size is Cohen's d. Cohen's d has the advantage of being widely reported, calculable from many common descriptive statistics, including some combination of F statistics, the number of subjects, means, standard errors and standard deviations.

Table 1 captures the basic information (Cohen, 2013) needed to calculate Cohen's d.

Table 1

Cohen's d Data Structure, Overview

	Group 1	Group 2
Mean	G1M	G2M
Standard Deviation	G1SD	G2SF
Sample Size (N)	G1N	G2N

The existence of two groups in Cohen's d means that such an approach cannot, without complex modifications, be used to compare effect sizes from more than two forms of dieting. The two-group structure of Cohen's d means that it is well-suited to comparing weight loss in a within-subjects model in which the two groups can be treated as matched pairs, with the 'before' state representing someone before embarking on a LCHF diet and the after state representing the same individual after a LCHF diet. Cohen's *d* can also be used to compare effect sizes across LCHF and non-LCHF groups. Table 2 offers an idea of how Cohen's *d* can be derived when making comparisons within an all-LCHF intervention; Table 3 demonstrates how Cohen's *d* can be calculated for LCHF and non-LCHF groups.

Table 2

Cohen's d Data Structure, All-LCHF Intervention

Individual	Weight Before LCHF Diet	Weight After LCHF Diet
1	*a*	*x*
2	*b*	*y*
3	*c*	*z*

To calculate Cohen's *d*, the data from Table 2 would be used to calculate a mean, standard deviation, and sample size for each column. This information could then be placed into an automated Cohen's *d* calculator (IDP, 2016) to calculate the effect size. The resulting effect size would be a control-intervention-based estimate of the effectiveness of an LCHF diet in the absence of other diets types to compare. This structure can be easily modified to accommodate studies in which LCHF and non-LCHF diet effects were provided. Such a structure has been provided in Table 3 below.

Table 3

Cohen's d Data Structure, Mixed Intervention

Individual	Weight Before LCHF Diet	Weight After LCHF Diet
#1 (LCHF)	*a*	*u*
#2 (LCHF)	*b*	*v*
#3 (LCHF)	*c*	*w*
#4 (Non-LCHF)	*d*	*x*
#5 (Non-LCHF)	*e*	*y*
#6 (Non-LCHF)	*f*	*z*

Using the approach in Table 3, Group 1 would consist of all individuals with the LCHF diet as an intervention; whereas, Group 2 would consist of all individuals with a diet other than the LCHF diet as an intervention. In such an approach, the means, standard deviations, and sample sizes would be calculated separately for Groups 1 and 2, and the results would be used to calculate Cohen's *d*. Note that this approach can be modified to

9

calculate the Cohen's *d* of a study in which some individuals are assigned to an LCHF diet group and other individuals comprise a control group.

Cohen's *d* was chosen as the measurement of effect size for this statistical meta-analysis. Cohen's *d* was chosen because it is both common and simple to calculate, on the basis of data structures such as those presented in Tables 1, 2, and 3 above. However, it should be noted that Cohen's *d* has some important limitations. In particular, Cohen's *d* is not well-suited to calculate effect sizes for studies in which there are two groups (such as an LCHF and non-LCHF group) and two experimental states (such as a control and an intervention group). The effect size measurement of Morris's *d* was created specifically for this situation). The absence of Morris's *d* and other more advanced forms of effect size calculation can be considered one of the limitations of the present study. However, given that many of the studies discussed and used as the basis of analysis, do not use advanced designs, the absence of Morris *d* calculations might not necessarily be a limitation of this study.

Having settled on Cohen's *d* as a measure of effect size, it is also necessary to discuss possible approaches to pooling. The simplest of all approaches is simply to average the Cohen's *d* sizes and to use the result as an estimate (Cohen, 2013). In more complex approaches (Cohen, 2013), effect sizes from different studies are accorded different weights based on factors such as the quality of the study, which could include level of evidence, participant size, and other factors. In this study, simple weighted averaging was used.

It should also be noted that all but three of the 12 studies included in this meta-analysis were meta-analyses. All meta-analyses report effect sizes. However, some meta-analyses do not report the Cohen's *d* effect size. For this reason, it was necessary to calculate Cohen's *d* based on the descriptive (and, in some cases, inferential) statistics reported in the meta-analyses and, where applicable, in the primary research articles.

Some interpretation of the range and meaning of Cohen's *d* values should also be provided. Cohen's *d* ranges from -3 to 3, with a score of 0 indicating the presence of 100% overlap between the two comparison groups. In the context of the study, the practical interpretation of a Cohen's *d* score of 0 would be that there is no difference between the weight loss of someone on an LCHF diet and someone not on a diet at all. A Cohen's *d* score of 3 would indicate that 100% of the treatment group (for example, the group on the LCHF diet) is above the mean of the control group (for example, the group not on the LCHF diet). Finally, a Cohen's *d* score of -3 would indicate that 100% of the treatment group is below the mean of the control group. Thus, a positive Cohen's *d* score would indicate the superiority of the LCHF diet vis-à-vis whatever it was compared diet.

Findings and Discussion

Table 4 below contains the overview of the 12 studies included in the statistical meta-analysis. Each study is described in terms of population, intervention, comparators, and outcome. In addition, each study is accompanied by both a Cohen's d value and a level of statistical significance, p. The values in the Cohen's d column were the values that were averaged to create a simple estimate of effect size, this is illustrated in Table 4.

Table 4

Table of Studies

Study	Population	Study Type	Intervention	Comparators	Outcome	N	p	Cohen's d (LCHF alone)	Cohen's d (non-LCHF)
Boaz et al. (2015)	American adults	Meta-Analysis	Dietary change	Low-fat diet	Weight loss	1161	< 0.05	0.56	0.41
Bueno et al. (2013)	American adults	Meta-Analysis	Dietary change	Low-fat diet Very low carb. Diet	Weight loss	1257	< 0.05	0.41	0.23
Clifton et al. (2014)	American adults	Meta-Analysis	Dietary change	None	Weight loss	3492	< 0.05	0.24	--
Franz et al. (2015)	American adults	Meta-Analysis	Dietary change	High-carb.	Weight loss	6754	< 0.05	0.82	0.19
Hooper et al. (2012)	American adults	Meta-Analysis	Dietary change	Low-fat	Weight loss	73589	< 0.05	1.01	0.76
Tian Hu et al. (2012)	American adults	Meta-Analysis	Dietary change	Low fat	Weight loss	2788	< 0.05	0.75	0.55
Ruth et al. (2013)	American adults	Clinical Trial	Dietary change	None	Weight loss	55	< 0.05	0.69	--
Santos et al. (2012)	American adults	Meta-analysis	Dietary change	None	Weight loss	1141	< 0.05	0.56	--
Soltani et	American	Meta-	Dietary	DASH diet	Weight	2206	< 0.05	0.11	0.09

al. (2016)	adults	analysis	change		loss				
Tobias et al. (2015)	American adults	Meta-analysis	Dietary change	Low-fat	Weight loss	68128	< 0.05	0.04	0.08
Tonstad et al. (2013)	American adults	Clinical Trial	Dietary change	Low-carb.	Weight loss	173	< 0.05	0.71	0.23
Wycherley et al. (2013)	American adults	Clinical Trial	Dietary change	Low-carb	Weight loss	56	< 0.05	0.50	0.10

Effect Size Calculations

The effect size calculations based on Table 4 indicated that the mean effect size for LCHF diets was higher ($M = 0.5333$, $SD = 0.29209$) than the mean effect size for non-LCHF diets at an Alpha of 0.10, $p = 0.058$. Where control group data for LCHF intervention groups were available, it was discovered that the mean effect size for LCHF diets ($M = 0.5333$, $SD = 0.29209$) in comparison to control (non-diet) groups ($M = 0.0358$, $SD = 0.03470$), $p < 0.001$ was also significantly greater.

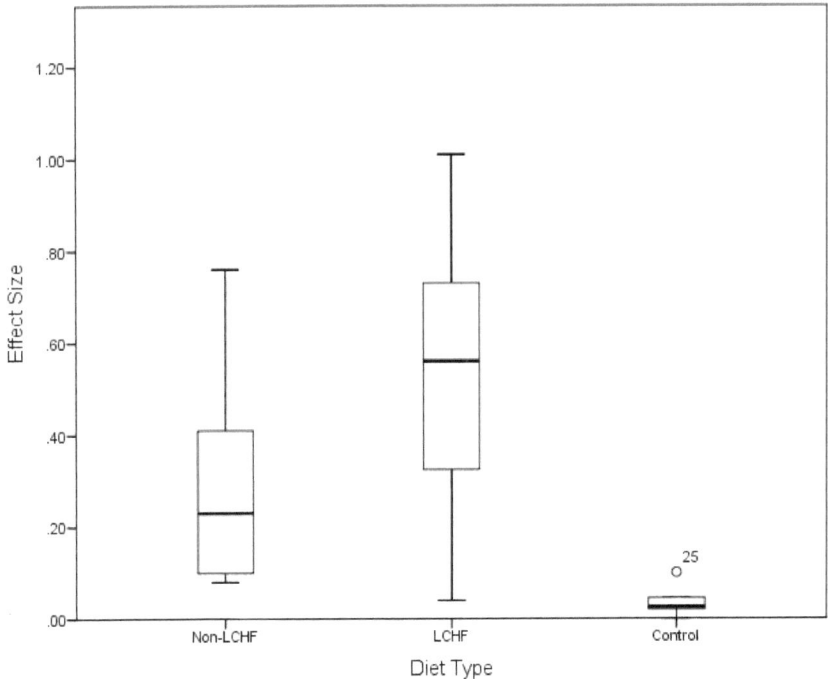

Figure 2. Boxplot of effect sizes by diet type.

The use of independent samples *t*-tests, results of which have been reported above and are visualized in the boxplot in Figure 2, support the conclusion that the LCHF diet had a greater effect size on weight loss. The boxplot in Figure 2, illustrates the significant increase in weight loss for the participants of the LCHF group, in relation to those participants in the non-LCHF and control groups. In fact, the lower quartile of the LCHF group is nearly equal to the upper quartile to the non-LCHF group.

Limitations

One of the study's limitations is an innate lack of statistical analysis. This limitation is best described through Roodman's (2007) discussion of Leamers'(1983) work. In discussing statistically-oriented scholarly work, Roodman stated that"

These papers differ not only in their conclusions but in their specifications as well…Although probably none of the choices are made on a whim; these differences appear to be examples of what Leamer called "whimsy." From Leamer's point of view

13

the studies together represent a small sampling of specification space. And few include much robustness testing. Without further analysis, it is hard to know whether the results reveal solid underlying regularities in the data or are fragile artifacts of particular specification choices. (Roodman, 2007).

The concept of limited specification space is particularly applicable to the empirical literature on LCHF diets. For example, even the definition of an LCHF diet is controversial, as there is no specific percentage of either carbohydrate consumption or fat consumption universally accepted as part of an LCHF. Because of the variability in different definitions of low-carbohydrate and high-fat components of an LCHF, the results of an effect size pooling based on such data are more likely to be fragile. The fragility exists not only because of variability in the macronutrient percentages but also because of the absence of isocaloric consumption in the empirical literature. If, for example, the effects of the number of grams of carbohydrates or fat on satiety vary by the number of calories consumed, or by the ratio of calories consumed to total daily energy expenditure, then meta-analytical comparison might also suffer from fragility. Unfortunately, in the absence of data from clinical trials that include metabolic wards and 6-month isolation periods—trials that do not exist, in any appreciable number, in the current body of evidence—it is difficult to conduct a statistical meta-analysis of the effect of LCHF diets on weight loss without risking fragility.

Discussion of Findings with Respect to Theory and Empirical Research

The main findings of the study were that (a) there is a statistically significant effect of LCHF diets on weight loss and that (b) the effect of LCHF diets is significantly greater weight loss than that of non-LCHF diets. These findings are in compliance with the governing law of energy balance, which states that weight loss is an effect of consuming fewer calories than are expended. None of the studies reviewed in the empirical analysis provided any evidence that conflicted with the energy balance law. In all cases, regardless of which diet was used, weight loss was imputed to the creation of an energy imbalance in which fewer calories were ingested than expended.

The finding related to the superior effect size of LCHF diets offer some support for the three explanatory physiological states identified, namely the state of general satiety (Berti et al., 2015; Fallaize et al., 2013; Gibbons et al., 2016), the switch to a fat-burning metabolism (Gillen et al., 2013; Liepinsh et al., 2014), and the way in which micronutrient and macronutrient consumption changes related to the adoption of an LCHF diet might also influence satiety (Horvath et al., 2014; Panagopoulou et al., 2014; Prentice, 2006; Tanumihardjo et al., 2007; Wells, 2012, 2013; Zapatero et al., 2013). The results of the

14

statistical meta-analysis provide empirical support for each of these explanatory physiological states. However, in the absence of additional measurement techniques, the effects of the LCHF diet on weight loss cannot be incontestably attributed to these three factors. For such conclusions to be drawn, more rigorous studies would have to be conducted, as described in the suggestions for future studies that follow.

Conclusion

Given the extent and vast public health and economic costs of the obesity epidemic (Frederick et al., 2014; Karp et al., 2014; Kay & McLaughlin, 2014; McClements, 2015; Pulgaron & Delamater, 2014; Sautkina et al., 2014; Shelton & Knott, 2014; Sieber et al., 2014; Tsai et al., 2014; Zilanawala et al., 2015; Zukiewicz-Sobczak et al., 2014), there is a substantial public interest in trying to measure the effectiveness of certain kinds of diets. However, evaluating the success of diets is an enormously complex procedure, because, outside of a strictly controlled environment (such as a metabolic ward), and without access to other reliable measurement tools, the results of a study could be less than definitive. Therefore, the most pressing problem confronting future researchers is how to collect and analyze the appropriate data, and perform such research in a strictly controlled environment, thus limiting the variables, and producing definitive results.

Recommendations

There is a need for further LCHF experimental research. In regard to a strictly controlled environment for this research, there are millions of inpatients in hospitals, and many of these inpatients are already exposed to calorie-controlled environments as part of treatment plans. This could be an opportunity to work directly with hospitals to create isocaloric meal plans with different macronutrient compositions and subsequently track weight loss. One limitation of such an approach is that dietary compliance would not be tested, as participants would have their food chosen for them. The advantage of such an environment would be the ability to measure the relationship between different macronutrient balances and involuntary calorie consumption. If it is found that an LCHF diet strategy is correlated with lower ad libitum calorie consumption, and that LCHF strategies are highly complied with, then there would be substantial evidence as to both how and why LCHF diets work.

The methods described above are statistical and correlational in nature, and, as such, they do not provide insight into an important component of dietary success, namely hormones. There is substantial evidence for the proposition that hormones are released or withheld in response to changes in diet, such that, for example, appetite is sharpened by

15

ghrelin, thus making hunger a hard state to sustain. It would be highly useful for future researchers to consider the differential effects of diets such as LCHF on hormonal systems, given that hormones are connected to appetite and homoeostasis.

LCHF diets are part of a matrix of approaches to the underlying problem, which is that of obesity. There are numerous methods for remediation of obesity, from the research studies used in this meta-analysis in the remediation of obesity. Four of these methods are described below:

- The promotion of diet-related behavioral change (Capacci et al., 2012; H. Peters et al., 2012; Reilly, J., 2012; Sautkina et al., 2014; Shelton & Knott, 2014; Zilanawala et al., 2015) by sponsoring advertisements and other marketing initiatives designed to encourage people, particularly children, to eat in a more healthy fashion.

- Targeted censorship (Capacci et al., 2012; H. Peters et al., 2012; J. J. Reilly, 2012; Sautkina et al., 2014; Shelton & Knott, 2014; Zilanawala et al., 2015) of advertising of highly calorific food, particularly in a context that would allow children to see such advertisements.

- The promotion of exercise-related behavioral change (Capacci et al., 2012; H. Peters et al., 2012; Reilly, 2012; Sautkina et al., 2014; Shelton & Knott, 2014; Zilanawala et al., 2015) by funding and providing other kinds of support for exercise programs in schools.

- Use of the medical industry to promote medical support for individuals with obesity, up to and including the provision of gastric bypass surgery (Capacci et al., 2012; H. Peters et al., 2012; Reilly, 2012; Sautkina et al., 2014; Shelton & Knott, 2014; Zilanawala et al., 2015)

Within this matrix of public health approaches, LCHF diets fit within the category of diet-related behavioral changes. The evidence presented in this statistical meta-analysis indicates that LCHF diets exert a substantial effect on weight loss, which in turn suggests that LCHF diets should be more heavily promoted than they currently are. However, this recommendation raises important questions about policy and practice that need to be considered carefully.

There is a consensus in the literature (Anderson & Butcher, 2006; CDC, 2014; Colagiuri, 2010; Deckelbaum & Williams, 2001; Evans, 2010; Koplan, Liverman, & Kraak, 2005; Lindelof, Nielsen, & Pedersen, 2011; Malterud & Ulriksen, 2010; NPR, 2012; Tsai et al., 2014; Zukiewicz-Sobczak et al., 2014) on obesity, that obesity is the result of a complex interaction of factors, including (a) the so-called obesogenic environment, one that is characterized by the absence of opportunities for exercise and the prevalence of sources of fast food and other forms of calorific food; (b) the conscious efforts of food companies to engineer highly calorific foods that are easy to overconsume; (c) the ineffectiveness of government's laissez faire approach to issues of food and health policy; and (d) individual food consumers' lack of knowledge, or motivation to commit to, certain forms of healthy eating. Given the complicated context of obesity itself, the role of government must be considered with caution. With obesity being a multi-factorial, complicated result, the entire responsibility for obesity cannot, and should not, be devolved on to public health policy (Bell, 2012; Colagiuri, 2010Dixon et al., 2005; Duncan, Magnuson, Kalil, & Ziol-Guest, 2012; Farag & Gaballa, 2011; Mason, Leavitt, & Chaffee, 2013; Schmidt & Duncan, 2003). As such, it would be inappropriate to suggest that an official promotion of LCHF diets would be either effective or warranted. Moreover, in the United States, the existence of a Food Pyramid reflects a consensus that a moderate-carbohydrate diet is healthy; it is unlikely that this consensus will be overturned by the evidence for the effectiveness of an LCHF diet. Nonetheless, the effect size of LCHF diets on weight loss demonstrated in this statistical meta-analysis could still inform both public and private efforts to inform consumers about healthier ways of eating.

The effect of an LCHF diet on weight loss among non-hospitalized American adults as measured after a minimum of 6 months, was answered in two complementary ways and both drew upon the Cohen's *d* measure of effect size. These findings provide empirical support for the claim that LCHF diets are effective, both in isolation and in comparison to other dietary interventions. These findings should be used as justification by private and public entities that wish to promote, within available institutional and other constraints, the adoption of LCHF diets among the public.

References

Anderson, P. M., & Butcher, K. F. (2006). Childhood obesity: trends and potential causes. *The Future of Children, 16*(1), 19-45. http://dx.doi.org/10.1353/foc.2006.0001

Bandini, L. G., Schoeller, D. A., Cyr, H. N., & Dietz, W. H. (1990). Validity of reported energy intake in obese and nonobese adolescents. *The American Journal of Clinical Nutrition, 52*(3), 421-425. Retrieved from http://ajcn.nutrition.org/content/52/3/421.full.pdf+html

Bell, E. (2012). *Research for health policy.* New York, NY: Oxford University Press. http://dx.doi.org/10.1093/acprof:oso/9780199549337.001.0001

Benedict, C., Axelsson, T., Söderberg, S., Larsson, A., Ingelsson, E., Lind, L., & Schiöth, H. B. (2014). Fat mass and obesity-associated gene (FTO) is linked to higher plasma levels of the hunger hormone ghrelin and lower serum levels of the satiety hormone leptin in older adults. *Diabetes, 63*(11), 3955-3959. http://dx.doi.org/10.2337/db14-0470

Berti, C., Riso, P., Brusamolino, A., & Porrini, M. (2015). Benefits of breakfast meals and pattern of consumption on satiety-related sensations in women. *International Journal of Food Sciences and Nutrition, 66*(7), 837-844. http://dx.doi.org/10.3109/09637486.2015.1093611

Black, A. E., Prentice, A. M., Goldberg, G. R., Jebb, S. A., Bingham, S. A., Livingstone, M. B. E., & Coward, A. (1993). Measurements of total energy expenditure provide insights into the validity of dietary measurements of energy intake. *Journal of the American Dietetic Association, 93*(5), 572-579. http://dx.doi.org/10.1016/0002-8223(93)91820-G

Boaz, M., Raz, O., & Wainstein, J. (2015). Low fat vs. low carbohydrate diet strategies for weight reduction: a meta-analysis. *Journal of Obesity & Weight Loss Therapy, 5*(273), 1. http://dx.doi.org/10.4172/2165-7904.1000273

Bowman, S., Clemens, J., Friday, J., & Moshfegh, A. (2016). The consumption of added sugars and solid fats by children, ages 12 to 19 years, reduced substantially in the United States from 2003-04 to 2011-12. *Journal of Nutrition Education and Behavior, 48*(7), S39. http://dx.doi.org/10.1016/j.jneb.2016.04.106

Brinkworth, G. D., Wycherley, T. P., Noakes, M., Buckley, J. D., & Clifton, P. M. (2016). Long-term effects of a very-low-carbohydrate weight-loss diet and an isocaloric low-fat diet on bone health in obese adults. *Nutrition, 32*(9), 1033-1036. http://dx.doi.org/10.1016/j.nut.2016.03.003

Bueno, N. B., de Melo, I. S. V., de Oliveira, S. L., & da Rocha Ataide, T. (2013). Very-low-carbohydrate ketogenic diet v. low-fat diet for long-term weight loss:A meta-analysis of randomised controlled trials. *British Journal of Nutrition, 110*(07), 1178-1187. https://doi.org/10.1017/S0007114513000548

Buhl, K. M., Gallagher, D., Hoy, K., Matthews, D. E., & Heymsfield, S. B. (1995). Unexplained disturbance in body weight regulation: diagnostic outcome assessed by doubly labeled water and body composition analyses in obese patients reporting low energy intakes. *Journal of the*

American Dietetic Association, 95(12), 1393-1400. http://dx.doi.org/10.1016/S0002-8223(95)00367-3

Campbell, D. T. (1988). *Methodology and epistemology for social sciences: Selected papers.* Chicago, IL: University of Chicago Press. Retrieved from https://books.google.com/books?hl=en&lr=&id=cLi-iz_8pYgC&oi=fnd&pg=PR7&dq=Methodology+and+epistemology+for+social+sciences&ots=ObfJ5kjmpv&sig=sP003U2oaaxd2F329FbtnlF23Vw#v=onepage&q=Methodology%20and%20epistemology%20for%20social%20sciences&f=false

Capacci, S., Mazzocchi, M., Shankar, B., Macias, J. B., Verbeke, W., Pérez-Cueto, F. J., . . . D'Addesa, D. (2012). Policies to promote healthy eating in Europe:A structured review of policies and their effectiveness. *Nutrition Reviews, 70*(3), 188-200. https://doi.org/10.1111/j.1753-4887.2011.00442.x

Centers for Disease Control and Prevention. (2014). Childhood obesity facts. Retrieved from http://www.cdc.gov/healthyyouth/obesity/facts.htm

Chambers, L., McCrickerd, K., & Yeomans, M. R. (2015). Optimising foods for satiety. *Trends in Food Science & Technology, 41*(2), 149-160. http://dx.doi.org/10.1016/j.tifs.2014.10.007

Clifton, P. M., Condo, D., & Keogh, J. B. (2014). Long term weight maintenance after advice to consume low carbohydrate, higher protein diets–a systematic review and meta analysis. *Nutrition, Metabolism and Cardiovascular Diseases, 24*(3), 224-235. http://dx.doi.org/10.1016/j.numecd.2013.11.006

Cochrane, A. L. (1972). *Effectiveness and efficiency.* Nuffield, U.K.: The Nuffield Provincial Hospitals Trust. Retrieved from https://www.nuffieldtrust.org.uk/research/effectiveness-and-efficiency-random-reflections-on-health-services

Cohen, J. (2013). *Statistical power analysis for the behavioral sciences.* New York, NY: Routledge. Retrieved from http://www.sciencedirect.com/science/book/9780121790608

Colagiuri, S. (2010). Diabesity: therapeutic options. *Diabetes, Obesity and Metabolism, 12*(6), 463-473. http://dx.doi.org/10.1111/j.1463-1326.2009.01182.x

Cooper, H., Hedges, L. V., & Valentine, J. C. (2009). *The handbook of research synthesis and meta-analysis.* New York, NY: Russell Sage Foundation. Retrieved from http://www.jstor.org/stable/10.7758/9781610441384

Cooper, J. A., Stevenson, J. L., & Paton, C. M. (2016). Hunger and satiety responses to saturated fat-rich meals before and after a high PUFA diet. *The FASEB Journal, 30*(1 Supplement), 405-407. http://dx.doi.org/10.1002/oby.21202

Crino, M., Sacks, G., Vandevijvere, S., Swinburn, B., & Neal, B. (2015). The influence on population weight gain and obesity of the macronutrient composition and energy density of the food supply. *Current Obesity Reports, 4*(1), 1-10. http://dx.doi.org/10.1007/s13679-014-0134-7

Deckelbaum, R. J., & Williams, C. L. (2001). Childhood obesity: The health issue. *Obesity Research, 9*(S11), 239-243. http://dx.doi.org/10.1038/oby.2001.125

Dickson, R., & Cherry, M. G. (2014). Defining my review question and identifying inclusion criteria. In R. Dickson, M. G. Cherry, & A. Boland (Eds.), *Doing a systematic review: A student's guide* (pp. 17-34). London, U.K.: Sage. Retrieved from http://eprints.lse.ac.uk/57308/

Dixon, J. B., Pories, W. J., O'Brien, P. E., Schauer, P. R., & Zimmet, P. (2005). Surgery as an effective early intervention for diabesity: why the reluctance? *Diabetes Care, 28*(2), 472-474. Retrieved from http://care.diabetesjournals.org/content/diacare/28/2/472.full.pdf

Duncan, G. J., Magnuson, K., Kalil, A., & Ziol-Guest, K. (2012). The importance of early childhood poverty. *Social Indicators Research, 108*(1), 87-98. Retrieved from https://www.researchgate.net/profile/Greg_Duncan3/publication/251190384_The_Importance _of_Early_Childhood_Poverty/links/57dff7e608ae1a73a5e389fb.pdf

Evans, B. (2010). Anticipating fatness: childhood, affect and the pre-emptive 'war on obesity'. *Transactions of the Institute of British Geographers, 35*(1), 21-38. http://dx.doi.org/10.1111/j.1475-5661.2009.00363.x

Faith, M. S., Heo, M., Kral, T. V., & Sherry, B. (2013). Compliant eating of maternally prompted food predicts increased body mass index z-score gain in girls: results from a population-based sample. *Childhood Obesity, 9*(5), 427-436. Retrieved from http://online.liebertpub.com/doi/10.1089/chi.2012.0098

Fallaize, R., Wilson, L., Gray, J., Morgan, L. M., & Griffin, B. A. (2013). Variation in the effects of three different breakfast meals on subjective satiety and subsequent intake of energy at lunch and evening meal. *European Journal of Nutrition, 52*(4), 1353-1359. http://dx/doi.org/10.1007/s00394-012-0444-z

Farag, Y. M., & Gaballa, M. R. (2011). Diabesity: an overview of a rising epidemic. *Nephrology Dialysis Transplantation, 26*(1), 28-35. https://doi.org/10.1093/ndt/gfq576

Franz, M. J., Boucher, J. L., Rutten-Ramos, S., & VanWormer, J. J. (2015). Lifestyle weight-loss intervention outcomes in overweight and obese adults with type 2 diabetes: a systematic review and meta-analysis of randomized clinical trials. *Journal of the Academy of Nutrition and Dietetics, 115*(9), 1447-1463. http://dx.doi.org/10.1016/j.jand.2015.02.031

Frederick, C. B., Snellman, K., & Putnam, R. D. (2014). Increasing socioeconomic disparities in adolescent obesity. *Proceedings of the National Academy of Sciences, 111*(4), 1338-1342. http://dx.doi.org/10.1073/pnas.1321355110

Fumagalli, M., Moltke, I., Grarup, N., Racimo, F., Bjerregaard, P., Jørgensen, M. E., . . . Linneberg, A. (2015). Greenlandic Inuit show genetic signatures of diet and climate adaptation. *Science, 349*(6254), 1343-1347. http://dx.doi.org/10.1126/science.aab2319

Gibbons, C., Caudwell, P., Finlayson, G., Webb, D.-L., Hellström, P. M., Näslund, E., & Blundell, J. E. (2013). Comparison of postprandial profiles of ghrelin, active GLP-1, and total PYY to meals varying in fat and carbohydrate and their association with hunger and the phases of satiety. *The Journal of Clinical Endocrinology & Metabolism, 98*(5), E847-E855. http://dx.doi.org/10.1210/jc.2012-3835

Gibbons, C., Finlayson, G., Caudwell, P., Webb, D.-L., Hellström, P. M., Näslund, E., & Blundell, J. E. (2016). Postprandial profiles of CCK after high fat and high carbohydrate meals and the relationship to satiety in humans. *Peptides, 77,* 3-8. http://dx.doi.org/10.1016/j.peptides.2015.09.010

Gibson, A., Seimon, R., Lee, C., Ayre, J., Franklin, J., Markovic, T., . . . Sainsbury, A. (2015). Do ketogenic diets really suppress appetite? A systematic review and meta-analysis. *Obesity Reviews, 16*(1), 64-76. http://dx.doi.org/10.1111/obr.12230

Gillen, J. B., Percival, M. E., Ludzki, A., Tarnopolsky, M. A., & Gibala, M. (2013). Interval training in the fed or fasted state improves body composition and muscle oxidative capacity in overweight women. *Obesity, 21*(11), 2249-2255. http://dx.doi.org/10.1002/oby.20379

Gluck, M. E., Yahav, E., Hashim, S. A., & Geliebter, A. (2014). Ghrelin levels after a cold pressor stress test in obese women with binge eating disorder. *Psychosomatic Medicine, 76*(1), 74-79. http://dx.doi.org/10.1097/PSY.0000000000000018

Halford, J. C., & Harrold, J. A. (2012). Satiety-enhancing products for appetite control: science and regulation of functional foods for weight management. *Proceedings of the Nutrition Society, 71*(02), 350-362. https://doi.org/10.1017/S0029665112000134

Hill, B. R., Rolls, B. J., Roe, L. S., De Souza, M. J., & Williams, N. I. (2013). Ghrelin and peptide YY increase with weight loss during a 12-month intervention to reduce dietary energy density in obese women. *Peptides, 49,* 138-144. http://dx.doi.org/10.1016/j.peptides.2013.09.009

Hooper, L., Abdelhamid, A., Moore, H. J., Douthwaite, W., Skeaff, C. M., & Summerbell, C. D. (2012). Effect of reducing total fat intake on body weight: systematic review and meta-analysis of randomised controlled trials and cohort studies. *BMJ, 345,* e7666. https://doi.org/10.1136/bmj.e7666

Hopkins, M., Finlayson, G., Duarte, C., Whybrow, S., Ritz, P., Horgan, G., . . . Stubbs, R. (2016). Modelling the associations between fat-free mass, resting metabolic rate and energy intake in the context of total energy balance. *International Journal of Obesity, 40*(2), 312-318. http://dx.doi.org/10.1038/ijo.2015.155

Horvath, J. D. C., de Castro, M. L. D., Kops, N., Malinoski, N. K., & Friedman, R. (2014). Obesity coexists with malnutrition? Adequacy of food consumption by severely obese patients to dietary reference intake recommendations. *Nutricion Hospitalaria, 29*(2), 292-299. http://dx.doi.org/10.3305/nh.2014.29.2.7053

Hu, T., Mills, K. T., Yao, L., Demanelis, K., Eloustaz, M., Yancy, W. S., . . . Bazzano, L. A. (2012). Effects of low-carbohydrate diets versus low-fat diets on metabolic risk factors: a meta-analysis of randomized controlled clinical trials. *American Journal of Epidemiology, 176*(suppl 7), 44-54. http://dx.doi.org/10.1093/aje/kws264

Hu, T., Yao, L., Reynolds, K., Niu, T., Li, S., Whelton, P., . . . Bazzano, L. (2016). The effects of a low-carbohydrate diet on appetite: A randomized controlled trial. *Nutrition, Metabolism and Cardiovascular Diseases, 26*(6), 476-488. http://dx.doi.org/10.1016/j.numecd.2015.11.011

IDP. (2016). Effect sizes. Retrieved from http://www.psychometrica.de/effect_size.html

Jakubowicz, D., & Froy, O. (2013). Biochemical and metabolic mechanisms by which dietary whey protein may combat obesity and Type 2 diabetes. *The Journal of Nutritional Biochemistry, 24*(1), 1-5. http://dx.doi.org/10.1016/j.jnutbio.2012.07.008

Jaremka, L. M., Fagundes, C. P., Peng, J., Belury, M. A., Andridge, R. R., Malarkey, W. B., & Kiecolt-Glaser, J. K. (2015). Loneliness predicts postprandial ghrelin and hunger in women. *Hormones and Behavior, 70*, 57-63. http://dx.doi.org/10.1016/j.yhbeh.2015.01.011

Kaplan, H., Hill, K., Lancaster, J., & Hurtado, A. M. (2000). A theory of human life history evolution: diet, intelligence, and longevity. *Evolutionary Anthropology Issues News and Reviews, 9*(4), 156-185. http://dx.doi.org/10.1002/1520-6505(2000)9:4<156::AID-EVAN5>3.0.CO;2-7

Karp, S. M., Barry, K. M., Gesell, S. B., Po'e, E. K., Dietrich, M. S., & Barkin, S. L. (2014). Parental feeding patterns and child weight status for Latino preschoolers. *Obesity Research & Clinical Practice, 8*(1), 88-97. http://dx.doi.org/10.1016/j.orcp.2012.08.193

Kay, G. G., & McLaughlin, D. (2014). Relationship between obesity and driving. *Current Obesity Reports, 3*(3), 336-340. http://dx.doi.org/10.1016/j.tranpol.2011.03.008

Koplan, J. P., Liverman, C. T., & Kraak, V. I. (2005). Preventing childhood obesity: health in the balance. *Journal of the American Dietetic Association, 105*(1), 131-138. Retrieved from https://www.nap.edu/catalog/11015/preventing-childhood-obesity-health-in-the-balance

Lichtman, S. W., Pisarska, K., Berman, E. R., Pestone, M., Dowling, H., Offenbacher, E., . . . Heymsfield, S. B. (1992). Discrepancy between self-reported and actual caloric intake and exercise in obese subjects. *New England Journal of Medicine, 327*(27), 1893-1898. http://dx.doi.org/10.1056/NEJM199212313272701

Liepinsh, E., Makrecka, M., Kuka, J., Makarova, E., Vilskersts, R., Cirule, H., . . . Dambrova, M. (2014). The heart is better protected against myocardial infarction in the fed state compared to the fasted state. *Metabolism, 63*(1), 127-136. http://dx.doi.org/10.1016/j.metabol.2013.09.014

Lindelof, A., Nielsen, C. V., & Pedersen, B. D. (2011). Obesity stigma at home: A qualitative, longitudinal study of obese adolescents and their parents. *Childhood Obesity, 7*(6), 462-474. http://dx.doi.org/10.1089/chi.2011.0021

Malterud, K., & Ulriksen, K. (2010). "Norwegians fear fatness more than anything else"—A qualitative study of normative newspaper messages on obesity and health. *Patient Education and Counseling, 81*(1), 47-52. http://dx.doi.org/10.1016/j.pec.2009.10.022

Mason, D. J., Leavitt, J. K., & Chaffee, M. W. (2013). *Policy and politics in nursing and healthcare.* New York, NY: Elsevier Health Sciences.

McClements, D. J. (2015). Reduced-fat foods: the complex science of developing diet-based strategies for tackling overweight and obesity. *Advances in Nutrition: An International Review Journal, 6*(3), 338S-352S. http://dx.doi.org/10.3945/an.114.006999

McGraw, K. O., & Wong, S. (1992). A common language effect size statistic. *Psychological Bulletin, 111*(2), 361-365. Retrieved from http://core.ecu.edu/psyc/wuenschk/docs30/CL.pdf

Mitchell, S. E., Delville, C., Konstantopedos, P., Hurst, J., Derous, D., Green, C., . . . Promislow, D. E. (2015). The effects of graded levels of calorie restriction: II. Impact of short term calorie and protein restriction on circulating hormone levels, glucose homeostasis and oxidative stress in male C57BL/6 mice. *Oncotarget, 6*(27), 23213-23237. http://dx.doi.org/10.18632/oncotarget.4003

Morris, S. B. (2008). Estimating effect sizes from the pretest-posttest-control group designs. *Organizational Research Methods, 11*(2), 364-386. Retrieved from http://journals.sagepub.com/doi/pdf/10.1177/1094428106291059

National Public Radio. (2012). Controversy swirls around harsh anti-obesity ads. Retrieved from http://www.npr.org/2012/01/09/144799538/controversy-swirls-around-harsh-anti-obesity-ads

Panagopoulou, P., Fotoulaki, M., Nikolaou, A., & Nousia-Arvanitakis, S. (2014). Prevalence of malnutrition and obesity among cystic fibrosis patients. *Pediatrics International, 56*(1), 89-94. http://dx.doi.org/10.1111/ped.12214

Peters, H., Whincup, P. H., Cook, D. G., Law, C., & Li, L. (2012). Trends in blood pressure in 9 to 11-year-old children in the United Kingdom 1980–2008: the impact of obesity. *Journal of Hypertension, 30*(9), 1708-1717. http://dx.doi.org/10.1097/HJH.0b013e3283562a6b

Peters, H. P., Bouwens, E. C., Schuring, E. A., Haddeman, E., Velikov, K. P., & Melnikov, S. M. (2014). The effect of submicron fat droplets in a drink on satiety, food intake, and cholecystokinin in healthy volunteers. *European Journal of Nutrition, 53*(3), 723-729. http://dx.doi.org/10.1007/s00394-013-0576-9

Phillips, S. M. (2014). A brief review of higher dietary protein diets in weight loss: a focus on athletes. *Sports Medicine, 44*(2), 149-153. http://dx.doi.org/10.1007/s40279-014-0254-y

Poulsen, S. K., Due, A., Jordy, A. B., Kiens, B., Stark, K. D., Stender, S., . . . Larsen, T. M. (2014). Health effect of the New Nordic Diet in adults with increased waist circumference: a 6-mo randomized controlled trial. *The American Journal of Clinical Nutrition, 99*(1), 35-45. http://dx.doi.org/10.3945/ajcn.113.069393

Prentice, A. M. (2006). The emerging epidemic of obesity in developing countries. *International Journal of Epidemiology, 35*(1), 93-99. http://dx.doi.org/10.1093/ije/dyi272

Pulgaron, E. R., & Delamater, A. M. (2014). Obesity and type 2 diabetes in children: epidemiology and treatment. *Current Diabetes Reports, 14*(8), 1-12. http://dx.doi.org/10.1007/s11892-014-0508-y

Reilly, D., Neumann, D. L., & Andrews, G. (2015). Sex differences in mathematics and science achievement: A meta-analysis of National Assessment of Educational Progress assessments. *Journal of Educational Psychology, 107*(3), 645-662. http://dx.doi.org/10.1037/edu0000012

Reilly, J. J. (2012). Evidence-based obesity prevention in childhood and adolescence: critique of recent etiological studies, preventive interventions, and policies. *Advances in Nutrition: An International Review Journal, 3*(4), 636S-641S. http://dx.doi.org/10.3945/an.112.002014

Roodman, D. (2007). The anarchy of numbers: aid, development, and cross-country empirics. *The World Bank Economic Review, 21*(2), 255-277. https://doi.org/10.1093/wber/lhm004

Rosenthal, R. (1994). Parametric measures of effect size. In H. Cooper & L. V. Hedges (Eds.), *The handbook of research synthesis* (pp. 231-244). New York, NY: Sage. Retrieved from http://psych.wfu.edu/furr/EffectSizeFormulas.pdf

Ruth, M. R., Port, A. M., Shah, M., Bourland, A. C., Istfan, N. W., Nelson, K. P., . . . Apovian, C. M. (2013). Consuming a hypocaloric high fat low carbohydrate diet for 12weeks lowers C-reactive protein, and raises serum adiponectin and high density lipoprotein-cholesterol in obese subjects. *Metabolism, 62*(12), 1779-1787. http://dx.doi.org/10.1016/j.metabol.2013.07.006

Santos, F., Esteves, S., da Costa Pereira, A., Yancy Jr, W., & Nunes, J. (2012). Systematic review and meta-analysis of clinical trials of the effects of low carbohydrate diets on cardiovascular risk factors. *Obesity Reviews, 13*(11), 1048-1066. http://dx.doi.org/10.1111/j.1467-789X.2012.01021.x

Sarker, M. R., Franks, S., & Caffrey, J. (2013). Direction of post-prandial ghrelin response associated with cortisol response, perceived stress and anxiety, and self-reported coping and hunger in obese women. *Behavioural Brain Research, 257*, 197-200. http://dx.doi.org/10.1016/j.bbr.2013.09.046

Sautkina, E., Goodwin, D., Jones, A., Ogilvie, D., Petticrew, M., White, M., & Cummins, S. (2014). Lost in translation? Theory, policy and practice in systems-based environmental approaches to obesity prevention in the Healthy Towns programme in England. *Health & Place, 29*, 60-66. http://dx.doi.org/10.1016/j.healthplace.2014.05.006

Schmidt, M. I., & Duncan, B. B. (2003). Diabesity: an inflammatory metabolic condition. *Clinical Chemistry and Laboratory Medicine, 41*(9), 1120-1130. http://dx.doi.org/10.1515/CCLM.2003.174

Schneider, E. B. (2013). Inescapable hunger? Energy cost accounting and the costs of digestion, pregnancy, and lactation. *European Review of Economic History, 17*(3), 340-363. https://doi.org/10.1093/ereh/het011

Shelton, J. N., & Knott, S. C. (2014). Association between alcohol calorie intake and overweight and obesity in English adults. *American Journal of Public Health, 104*(4), 629-631. http://dx.doi.org/10.2105/AJPH.2013.301643

Sieber, W. K., Robinson, C. F., Birdsey, J., Chen, G. X., Hitchcock, E. M., Lincoln, J. E., . . . Sweeney, M. H. (2014). Obesity and other risk factors: The National Survey of US Long-Haul Truck Driver Health and Injury. *American Journal of Industrial Medicine, 57*(6), 615-626. http://dx.doi.org/10.1002/ajim.22293

Slining, M. M., & Popkin, B. M. (2012). Trends in sources of empty calories for 2–18 year olds in the US: 1977–2008. *The FASEB Journal, 26*(1), 256.252-256.252. http://dx.doi.org/10.1111/j.2047-6310.2013.00156.x

Soltani, S., Shirani, F., Chitsazi, M. J., & Salehi-Abargouei, A. (2016). The effect of dietary approaches to stop hypertension (DASH) diet on weight and body composition in adults: a systematic review and meta-analysis of randomized controlled clinical trials. *Obesity Reviews, 17*(5), 442-454. http://dx.doi.org/10.1111/obr.12391

Tanumihardjo, S. A., Anderson, C., Kaufer-Horwitz, M., Bode, L., Emenaker, N. J., Haqq, A. M., . . . Stadler, D. D. (2007). Poverty, obesity, and malnutrition: an international perspective recognizing the paradox. *Journal of the American Dietetic Association, 107*(11), 1966-1972. http://dx.doi.org/10.1016/j.jada.2007.08.007

Thalheimer, W., & Cook, S. (2002). How to calculate effect sizes from published research articles: A simplified methodology. *Work Learning Research.* Retrieved from http://www.bwgriffin.com/gsu/courses/edur9131/content/Effect_Sizes_pdf5.pdf

Thomas, D. M., Gonzalez, M. C., Pereira, A. Z., Redman, L. M., & Heymsfield, S. B. (2014). Time to correctly predict the amount of weight loss with dieting. *Journal of the Academy of Nutrition and Dietetics, 114*(6), 857-861. http://dx.doi.org/10.1016/j.jand.2014.02.003

Thomas, D. M., Martin, C. K., Lettieri, S., Bredlau, C., Kaiser, K., Church, T., . . . Heymsfield, S. B. (2013). Can a weight loss of one pound a week be achieved with a 3500-kcal deficit? Commentary on a commonly accepted rule. *International Journal of Obesity, 37*(12), 1611-1613. http://dx.doi.org/10.1038/ijo.2013.51

Thorburn, A. N., Macia, L., & Mackay, C. R. (2014). Diet, metabolites, and "western-lifestyle" inflammatory diseases. *Immunity, 40*(6), 833-842. http://dx.doi.org/10.1016/j.immuni.2014.05.014

Tobias, D. K., Chen, M., Manson, J. E., Ludwig, D. S., Willett, W., & Hu, F. B. (2015). Effect of low-fat diet interventions versus other diet interventions on long-term weight change in adults: a systematic review and meta-analysis. *The Lancet Diabetes & Endocrinology, 3*(12), 968-979. http://dx.doi.org/10.1016/S2213-8587(15)00367-8

Tonstad, S., Malik, N., & Haddad, E. (2014). A high-fibre bean-rich diet versus a low-carbohydrate diet for obesity. *Journal of Human Nutrition and Dietetics, 27*(s2), 109-116. http://dx.doi.org/10.1111/jhn.12118

Torgerson, C. (2004). *Systematic reviews.* New York, NY: A&C Black.

Tsai, A. G., Boyle, T. F., Hill, J. O., Lindley, C., & Weiss, K. (2014). Changes in obesity awareness, obesity identification, and self-assessment of health: results from a statewide public education campaign. *American Journal of Health Education, 45*(6), 342-350. http://dx.doi.org/10.1080/19325037.2014.945668

Vink, R. G., Roumans, N. J., Arkenbosch, L. A., Mariman, E., & van Baak, M. A. (2016). The effect of rate of weight loss on long-term weight regain in adults with overweight and obesity. *Obesity, 24*(2), 321-327. http://dx.doi.org/10.1002/oby.21346

Walsh, J. A. (2013). Obesity & the First Law of Thermodynamics. *The American Biology Teacher, 75*(6), 413-415. http://dx.doi.org/10.1525/abt.2013.75.6.10

Weijenberg, M. P., Hughes, L. A., Bours, M. J., Simons, C. C., van Engeland, M., & van den Brandt, P. A. (2013). The mTOR pathway and the role of energy balance throughout life in colorectal cancer etiology and prognosis: unravelling mechanisms through a multidimensional molecular epidemiologic approach. *Current Nutrition Reports, 2*(1), 19-26. http://dx.doi.org/10.1007/s13668-012-0038-7

Wells, J. C. (2012). Obesity as malnutrition: the role of capitalism in the obesity global epidemic. *American Journal of Human Biology, 24*(3), 261-276. http://dx.doi.org/10.1002/ajhb.22253

Wells, J. C. (2013). Obesity as malnutrition: the dimensions beyond energy balance. *European Journal of Clinical Nutrition, 67*(5), 507-512. http://dx.doi.org/10.1038/ejcn.2013.31

Westerterp-Plantenga, M. S., Lemmens, S. G., & Westerterp, K. R. (2012). Dietary protein–its role in satiety, energetics, weight loss and health. *British Journal of Nutrition, 108*(S2), S105-S112. http://dx.doi.org/10.1017/S0007114512002589

Wycherley, T. P., Buckley, J. D., Noakes, M., Clifton, P. M., & Brinkworth, G. D. (2013). Comparison of the effects of weight loss from a high-protein versus standard-protein energy-restricted diet on strength and aerobic capacity in overweight and obese men. *European Journal of Nutrition, 52*(1), 317-325. http://dx.doi.org/10.1007/s00394-012-0338-0

Wycherley, T. P., Luscombe-Marsh, N., Thompson, C., Buckley, J., Noakes, M., Wittert, G., & Brinkworth, G. (2014). Effects of weight loss with a very low carbohydrate, low saturated fat diet on endothelial function in patients with T2DM. *Journal of Nutrition & Intermediary Metabolism, 1*, 34-35. http://dx.doi.org/10.1016/j.atherosclerosis.2016.07.908

Zapatero, A., Barba, R., Ruiz, J., Losa, J., Plaza, S., Canora, J., & Marco, J. (2013). Malnutrition and obesity: influence in mortality and readmissions in chronic obstructive pulmonary disease patients. *Journal of Human Nutrition and Dietetics, 26*(1), 16-22. http://dx.doi.org/10.1111/jhn.12088

Zilanawala, A., Davis-Kean, P., Nazroo, J., Sacker, A., Simonton, S., & Kelly, Y. (2015). Race/ethnic disparities in early childhood BMI, obesity and overweight in the United Kingdom and United States. *International Journal of Obesity, 39*(3), 520-529. http://dx.doi.org/10.1038/ijo.2014.171

Zuk, M. (2013). *Paleofantasy: What evolution really tells us about sex, diet, and how we live.* New York, NY: WW Norton & Company. Retrieved from http://books.wwnorton.com/books/Paleofantasy/

Zukiewicz-Sobczak, W., Wroblewska, P., Zwoliński, J., Chmielewska-Badora, J., Adamczuk, P., Krasowska, E., . . . Silny, W. (2014). Obesity and poverty paradox in developed countries. *Annals of Agricultural and Environmental Medicine, 21*(3), 590-594. http://dx.doi.org/10.5604/12321966.1120608

Appendix A

Search strings used:

- "weight loss" AND "low-carbohydrate, high fat"
- "weight loss" AND "low-carbohydrate, high fat" AND "6 months"
- "fat loss" AND "low-carbohydrate, high fat"
- "fat loss" AND "low-carbohydrate, high fat diet" AND "6 months"
- "weight loss" AND "low-carbohydrate, high fat diet"
- "weight loss" AND "low-carbohydrate, high fat diet" AND "6 months"
- "fat loss" AND "low-carbohydrate, high fat diet"
- "fat loss" AND "low-carbohydrate, high fat diet" AND "6 months"
- "weight loss" AND "LCHF diet"
- "weight loss" AND "LCHF diet" AND "6 months"
- "fat loss" AND "LCHF diet"
- "fat loss" AND "LCHF diet" AND "6 months"

Appendix B

PRISMA flow diagram for statistical meta-analysis.

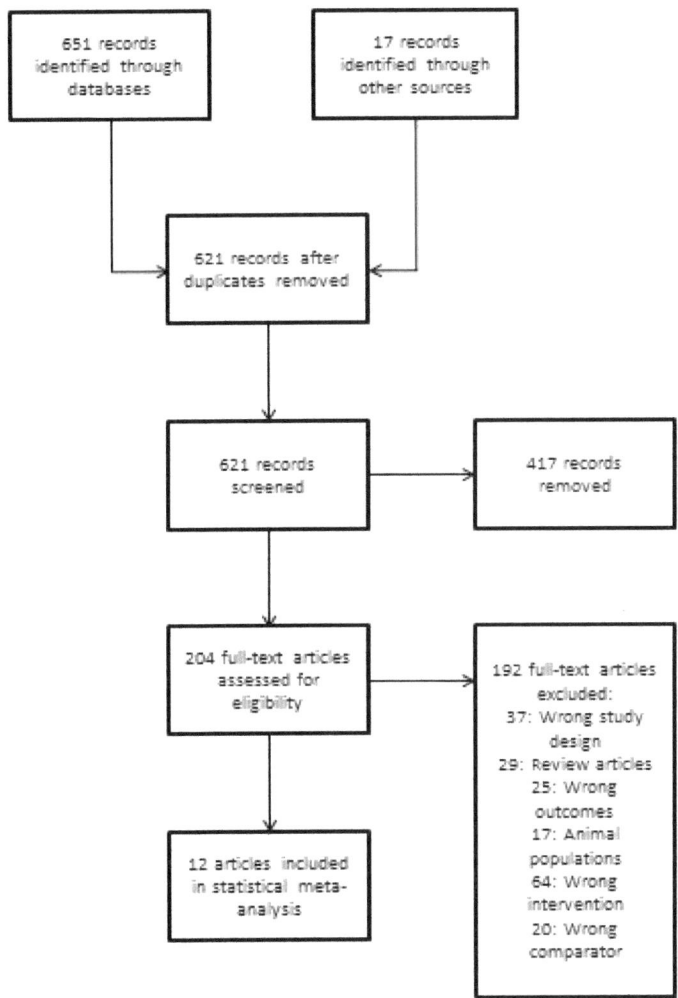

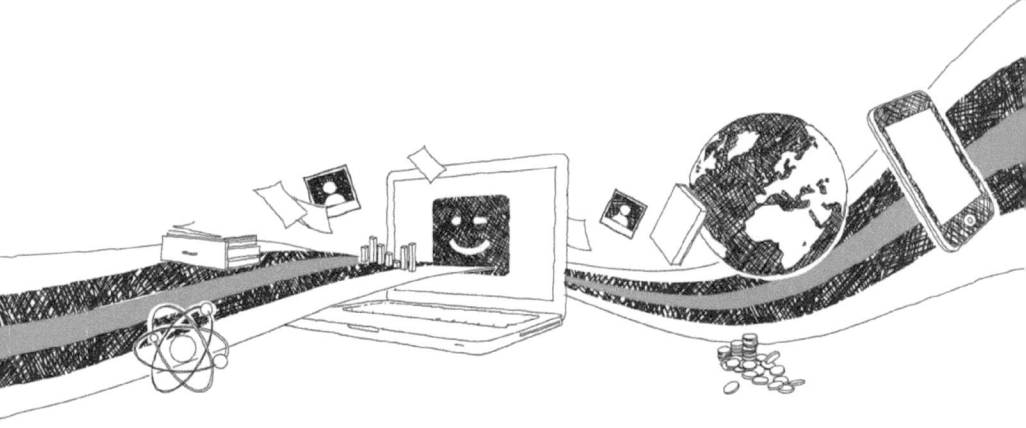
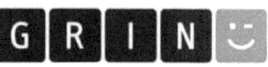